ACCOUNTABILITY
THE MISSING PIECE

KIMBERLY JOHNSON

ACCOUNTABILITY: *The Missing Piece*

Copyright© 2022 by Kimberly Johnson

All rights reserved. No part of this book may be reproduced or transmitted in any form or by any means without written permission from the author, except for brief quotations for reviews or articles.

Printed in the United States of America

Dedication:

To Mary Lou, my first accountability partner.
What a Godsend you are!

TABLE OF CONTENTS

INTRODUCTION 1

CHAPTER 1: How Accountability Changes Lives 4

CHAPTER 2: Accountability is God and People 11

CHAPTER 3: Accountability In Practice 22

CHAPTER 4: Sample Accountability Questions 37

CHAPTER 5: A Call to Action 43

EPILOGUE: Accountability Quotes 48

INTRODUCTION

For over 20 years, I was bound by destructive habits. I repeatedly tried to overcome them on my own, but I failed. I even went to a Christian counsellor and opened up about these things. Unfortunately, out of what she believed was protection for me, she told me not to tell anyone about my struggle. Her advice, although well-intended, was misguided. Because once I began to open up to people, everything changed. I started being accountable for my actions to others in my circle. Simply put, with accountability came freedom.

As a believer, I understand that most Christians know intuitively that accountability is helpful. However, I have found that few of them know how to walk it out in practical ways. This book is intended to help do that. I have seen accountability change the lives of hundreds of people that I have been blessed to walk with. It has changed my life, and it can change yours. I genuinely believe that accountability is the missing piece. The missing piece to what? Lasting change in *your* life!

Lord,

I thank You that the reader and I can take this journey together. It was for freedom that You set us free. I pray that the words on these pages would help the person reading them walk out the freedom in Christ that already belongs to them.

AMEN

CHAPTER 1

HOW ACCOUNTABILITY CHANGES LIVES

ACCOUNTABILITY: THE MISSING PIECE

It was another New Year's Eve, and I sat reflecting over the previous year while also thinking about the year to come. I was frustrated that another year had passed where I had not kept the promise I made to myself and God to stop my destructive habits. I took out a wall calendar for the next year and wrote across the top of January, "No More." I knew that no one else who saw the calendar would realize what I was talking about. But I knew exactly what I was talking about. No more of my destructive addictive habits that plagued me day after day, month after month, and year after year. I'm sad to say, that year did not conclude in the "No More" I professed over it.

A couple more years passed where I continued to try willpower, reading self-help books, staying busy, being secluded, fasting, praying, and almost every other spiritual discipline you could think of. So here I was, bound for over 20 years, desperate, and at the end of myself. I couldn't go on anymore, and I knew that things had to change. I felt the Lord leading me to open up to a friend, and I did. She set up some practical guidelines, and we entered into an accountability relationship. As a result, my life was changed forever.

Before I continue my story, because there are so many different ideas about accountability, I want to define accountability as it pertains to my brief testimony and the majority of this book (we will briefly discuss other components of accountability in chapter three). I'm specifically referring to the courage to invite someone alongside you to reach your goals. Daring to be honest, committing to checking in with them and letting them into this portion of your journey. Accountability is about utilizing another person to help us achieve what we desire or know we need to achieve. It is not something you have; it is something you do. It's giving an account and having someone to give it to. It's not about success or failure, but it's about growth. It's not about inviting someone to call us out on our behavior. It's about inviting someone to call us to the creature we already are in Christ. This is why accountability isn't just for someone who wants to stop a habit. It is for anyone who wants to accomplish a goal or grow in any way. When we talk about equity, we often immediately think of finances, but in my opinion, the best equity we can have is relational equity. Accountability is about drawing from that equity.

ACCOUNTABILITY: THE MISSING PIECE

So to continue with my story, I invited someone to come alongside me. Together, we came up with questions I would be responsible for answering about my habit. I knew that answering questions about whether or not I engaged in my habit wouldn't be enough. So, we also set up questions about what I would do when I was tempted. In addition, we set up questions for if I did yield - questions about what I was going to do better next time and what I did or didn't do that caused me to yield. We met once a week for about 6 months and went over questions about my emotional state and whether or not I was being deliberate about discipline in several areas. In addition to that, we checked in daily for 2 years, and I answered yes or no if I slipped. During the first couple of months, the Lord also had me add in my pastor and a counselor for additional accountability. It suddenly became very uncomfortable to succumb to these habits. At the time of this writing, I have over 16 years of freedom in this area. Since then, I've added accountability to help me develop good habits and goals and maintain my freedom from bad habits. Even this book is a result of accountability. I have accountability in weight loss, cleaning, organizing, time spent on entertainment, etc. Anytime I have an important goal to reach or habit to change, I know that accountability will be the difference-maker.

But don't just take my word for it, I'd like to share with you a couple of quotes from some clients and mentors regarding accountability.

"Accountability was the missing component in my path to freedom from addiction. I often felt that I had to battle my compulsions alone. Never realizing the stigma and shame from these behaviors kept me in an endless cycle of failure, shame, repentance, vowing to change, only to repeat the cycle all over again. When I learned about accountability, I was met with my own fears rising to the surface in anticipation of those I would let into my struggle abandoning me. To my surprise, accountability has led to freedom from that stigma of shame, as those who have come alongside me have been an anchor and support in my journey. I am now able to face the lie that you are alone; with the truth that I am indeed surrounded by those who cheer me on advocating for my recovery and freedom. I couldn't imagine going through a journey of healing and deliverance from addiction without accountability" - **Client A.**

"The thought of telling someone about my addiction was mortifying, to say the least. Having an ongoing confession session with someone even made me angry at times. I was full of fear about it. I didn't want to feel embarrassed. I felt ashamed; I cried, kicked, resisted, and refused. I didn't want to admit that I needed help. I wanted to be strong and in control, like I perceived 'they' were. I didn't want them to see me as weak or needy. It took me a while to do it. But as difficult as it was, I'm experiencing an incredible sense of freedom. I didn't die, they didn't run away from me, and they didn't tell me how bad I was. I also see James 5:16 in a new light, **"Confess your sins to one another and pray for one another that you may be healed."** I didn't realize it, but before this, I saw that as a suggestion or something I'm supposed to try because it might help. But now I see that being accountable to another person makes me feel freer. I don't have to hide anymore. I feel known. I can be truthful and open about my stuff, and it's okay. The issues that have plagued my life for so long are decreasing. I don't think these things would be happening without accountability" - **Client B**.

"I have been meeting with people for personal spiritual and leadership growth for over two decades. The people who found the most freedom and reached the goals they set the fastest were willing to be held accountable for their commitments. Perhaps what made a big difference for these clients is when they reframed the word accountability, with positive descriptions, it became a positive motivator" - Rob Stoppard, Personal Growth Specialist (destinyui.com)

"We all have heard ourselves say, 'I know what to do, I just need to do it. Accountability is the secret link that connects desires with action. Accountability is the underpinning of everything that we do." - Lindsay House, RD (healthaccountabilitycoach.com)

> **Question to ponder:**
>
> What goals could be achieved a year from now if I implemented this type of accountability today?

CHAPTER 2

ACCOUNTABILITY IS GOD AND PEOPLE

GOD:

If you don't want to just learn to white-knuckle it and instead want to be made whole, God must be a part of your recovery equation. Just to make it clear, I'm not talking about some sort of arbitrary higher power here. I'm talking about Jesus Christ, the God of the Bible. For Christians, the goal is to be transformed into His image, and we can't do that without Him.

"Yes, I am the vine, you are the branches. Those who remain in me and I in them, will produce much fruit. For apart from me, you can do nothing" (John 15:5 NLT).

If God says it's nothing, then it doesn't matter what the world says. It's nothing.

"How foolish can you be after starting your new lives in the spirit why are you now trying to become perfect by your own human effort?" (Galatians 3:3 NLT).

Although we have a part in our journey, it is not about willpower. Instead, it is about learning to implement God's power through us, and part of that is utilizing the resources He gave us, including people.

PEOPLE:

Self:

The first person we must be accountable to is ourselves. We can have everything in place as tools, ask God to help us, and even have an accountability partner. But if we aren't willing to take full responsibility, everything else will be fruitless. It isn't fair to ask someone else to work harder than we are willing to make positive changes in our lives. Not only is it unfair, it just simply won't work. It's not about making God or other people responsible for our changes. It's about utilizing them as gifts.

Others:

When I was in the heart of my recovery and healing, I had the following conversation with my counselor and mentor, Russell Willingham. (Because Russell is so wise in this area, I've asked him to write a little something, which will be shared at the end of this chapter).

Me: "Are you sure I'm being fair to God by involving others in this area of my life? Shouldn't He be enough?"

Russ: "Your journey of healing isn't God or people. It's God and people."

This conversation was transformational. I was reminded that every area of my spiritual journey involved God and people.

He used people to introduce me to Christ, He used people to help me grow in Christ, and this area would be no different. God and people. This is not about changing behavior. It's about changing our hearts. I am hoping for wholeness for you, which will involve utilizing God and people.

Even secular science, as is often the case, supports the truth of the need for people. For example, let's look at a study from the 1970s by American psychologist, Dr. Bruce Alexander. Alexander's experiments have come to be called "The Rat Park". Researchers during that time had already proved that when rats were placed in a cage all alone with no other community of rats and offered two water bottles, one filled with water only and the other with added heroin or cocaine, the rats would repeatedly drink from the drug-laced bottles until they all overdosed and died. They were relentless until their bodies and brains were overcome, and they died. I just want to say, although I'm not a proponent of animal or human experiments, I think as we continue, you will see the benefit of what was learned. Alexander wondered, "Is this about the drug, or about the environment they were in?"

To test his hypothesis, he put rats in "rat parks," where they were among others and free to roam and play, to socialize and to have sex. They were given the same access to the same two types of water bottles (one laced with drugs, one without). When inhabiting a Rat Park, they remarkably preferred the plain water. Even when they did drink from the drug-filled bottle, they did so intermittently, not obsessively, and never overdosed. Again, they *never* overdosed. A social community beat the power of drugs.

Only Jesus can provide forgiveness and ultimate healing. But we need others to be included in that healing. James 5:16 says, *"Confess your faults to one another and pray for one another that you may be healed."* Part of the healing process involves others. This scripture doesn't say to confess your faults to others so that you may be forgiven; it says so you may be healed. I don't want to just be set free from bad habits. I want to be free and healed from what led me to them in the first place. I don't just want to engage in healthy habits. I want the freedom of my life to reflect the freedom in my soul. How about you? Very often, addictions, bad habits, and trouble maintaining healthy habits result from brokenness. If we were broken, we would be healed and made whole in relationships.

"How important is accountability? I believe it is so important that there is neither recovery nor Christianity without it. How can I make such a bold statement? I base it on three things. Number one, I base it on my consistent experience (and many others) working with addicted people for three decades. Number two, I base it on the clear, unmistakable testimony of scripture. And, number three, I base it on my own experience of finding much healing and growth regarding my own brokenness over the years. Without accountability, people dealing with addictions and compulsive behaviors do not become well. By themselves, they can certainly improve; make behavioral changes, or "white knuckle" their way through sobriety for periods. But these are not the same as lasting change. And they certainly aren't the same as relational healing (the core need for every addict).

The crying need for every person who uses drinking, drugging, or acting out sexually to numb their pain is not simply to stop doing those things (though they do need to stop). The crying need is for them to find a heartfelt connection. For the addict, this begins with being accountable to another person (or persons) regarding their behaviors, but it cannot stop there. Real accountability must extend to the internal realm as well. When we share our thoughts, fears, hopes, motives, hidden agendas—even our deep ache for love- we are practicing accountability in its truest form. By this time, accountability has morphed into something else. It has become friendship, intimacy, love. We feel known and safe. This isn't romantic or sexual love. It's what the Bible calls "fellowship." Fellowship is a much bigger and richer experience than most Christians know. In Acts 2:44 we are told, "All the believers were together and had everything in common." This doesn't just mean they hung out and liked the same stuff. It means they were like one person and had the same heart. In other words: no barriers, no secrets, no posturing. Transparency. A few chapters later, we read that, "No one claimed that any of their possessions was their own, but they shared everything they had" (Acts 4:32). We make a big deal of how the early church took care of its own and how nobody went without (and that is a big deal). But the verse just before this explains why they did this, "All the believers were one in heart and mind." This is how deep, honest, and connected they were. Since their hearts were already completely open to each other, why wouldn't their bank accounts be as well? I've seen recovery groups, Sunday school classes, or tight-knit fellowships that were truly open, transparent, and loving with each other. And when a material need arose, that group got the resources together to meet the need. This didn't happen because they practiced "socialism"; it happened because they were accountable to each other and cared. Accountability is also the only thing standing between the addict and self-deception. Though we hate what our addictions do to us, we also love our addictions and will stop at nothing to protect them and keep them from being exposed (the double-minded person is unstable in all his ways – James 1:8). The Bible warns us about the constant danger of returning to our old, diseased way of thinking. In fact, scripture assumes that part of us is going in this direction all the time. Our heart naturally tends toward sin, unbelief, and turning away from God: "See to it, brothers and sisters, that none of you has a sinful, unbelieving heart that turns away from the living God." (Heb 3:12) This is a perfect description of the mental gymnastics we addicts do every day: denying the seriousness of our problems, justifying, rationalizing, minimizing our pain, blame-shifting, isolating, keeping secrets, being mad at God/the church/the world/ourselves, seeking comfort in our addiction instead of seeking comfort in God. With all of this deeply entrenched thinking inside us, what hope do we have of ever breaking free? The Bible tells us in the next verse: "But encourage one another daily, as long as it is called "Today," so that none of you may be hardened by sin's deceitfulness." (Heb 3:13) So what will turn the tide on a heart that tends toward growing hard and slipping back into self-deception? Only one thing—another person who stands in the way. We need someone who will encourage (exhort, call out to us, come alongside) us regularly. Of course, we can lie to them too if we want to. All accountability relationships are voluntary and covenantal. But accountability and close connected relationships (with Jesus and others) are God's means of getting us healthy. By the way, I have applied this verse to addicts (and it fits perfectly), but this verse in Hebrews is not spoken in a "recovery" context. It is spoken in a discipleship context. To say it another way, accountability isn't a recovery thing; it's a Bible thing. It's a Christian thing. I told you there was no Christianity without it. What about me? Do I practice what I preach? I have to. Not because I lead a recovery ministry but because I want to be healthy. My own addiction didn't budge until I told someone else. That person happened to be a Christian counselor. That was the beginning of life-change for me. I began to see what was deep inside me, and that gave me enough understanding to bring my true self to Jesus for healing. Since then, I have always had two to three people in my life who know me as well as my wife does (or better). I meet with them regularly. No subject is off-limits. In fact (especially in the early days), if one or both of us didn't feel terror at some point in the conversation, we knew we were probably hiding something. Are we blunt with each other? Yes. Do we also build each other up? We do that too. I discovered years ago that the addictive "need" I had was actually just a need for love. And—to my surprise—I started getting that need met by a couple of brothers. Of course, Jesus is the ultimate satisfier of my deepest need. Since I still have a bottomless need, I require a bottomless resource. But I was also created to be loved at a human level (to not "be alone," as God said in Genesis 2:18). A spouse is not enough to take away that "aloneness." I must have others like me who see me, know me and accept me at the deepest levels. Like Jesus (on whom I have to feed daily), I need two or three intimate friends that can help me belong continually. I will either fill my love tank in healthy ways or go back to my dumpster. How about you?" [1]

Now that we have spent a couple of chapters laying out the whys of accountability, let's spend some time on the hows!

> **Question to Ponder:**
>
> While keeping James 5:16 in mind, *"Confess your faults one to another and pray for one another, that you may be healed."* Ask yourself: What may still need healing in my life because I haven't involved others in my journey?

---

[1] © 2022 Russell Willingham, New Creation Ministries

CHAPTER 3

ACCOUNTABILITY IN PRACTICE

ACCOUNTABILITY: THE MISSING PIECE

I mentioned this in the previous chapter, but it is worth repeating. First and foremost, I have to be accountable for my own actions. Being accountable to another person or even God, for that matter, isn't going to make the difference if I don't honestly want to change. You don't have to be 100% willing to change a habit to have accountability, but you do at least need to be willing to be made willing. Accountability alone isn't going to make you want to change. It's something you add when you are ready to make changes. Good accountability is not just about changing your behavior; it's about changing your thinking.

Don't make the all too common mistake of opening up to someone and assuming that the other person will automatically follow up. What usually happens is the one opening up wants help, the one being opened up to wants to help, but neither one knows what steps to take and is waiting for the other to follow up. This is where many people get stuck. As mentioned previously, intuitively people know that accountability is a good thing but don't know how to practice it.

The most important thing that I've learned about accountability is that it can be simple, but it must be structured and detailed. It must be communicated clearly between both parties. If you tell the other party what you need instead of just opening up, it will give them the chance to tell you they can help or that they cannot. Don't get discouraged if someone tells you they are unable to commit. Being an accountability partner to someone is a big commitment. You would rather hear upfront that the person can't do it than find out in the middle of the process.

My goal for this chapter and the next is to help you practice the implementation of structured accountability, detail it and communicate it.

Remember, there is not necessarily a right or wrong way to do this. Accountability doesn't have to be perfect to work. But it doesn't work if it's not implemented.

This Chapter will discuss some of the most frequent ways that accountability is utilized: Accountability Partners, Apps/ Software, and Paid Accountability Coaches.

Accountability Partners:

Below are some of the most common questions I am asked about accountability.
1. **Why should I even have a partner?**

    Most people who asked this question have already tried to break free on their own, and they haven't been able to. To that I say, the definition of insanity is doing what you have always done and expecting a different result. If you could have done it on your own, you already would have. The Bible makes it very clear that two are better than one. One can put 1,000 to flight, two can put 10,000 to flight (See Deut 32:30). The Lord designed us to need one another. Having another person alongside you meets the need to be accountable, but more importantly, helps meet the need for love.

2. **Can I have a partner who struggles with the same issue as me, or do I need to have someone who doesn't?**

This is a question I get asked a lot, and it goes back to there's no right or wrong way to do it. For the most part, my accountability partners were people who did not struggle with the same things I did. Those were the available people, and those were the people God led me to. So, if you choose an accountability partner that struggles in the same way as you, I recommend additionally seeking someone out who doesn't struggle in the area you're trying to improve. Sometimes it's a little less comfortable to share with them that you had a slip than it would be sharing with a fellow struggler in that area. Part of the purpose of accountability is for it to be a deterrent by knowing it will be uncomfortable sharing if we sin or slip. Also, if you have someone who struggles in the same area as you, please make sure that the two of you are careful not to use triggering language with one another. To protect you both, brief descriptions, check-ins, and constant communication about what you will discuss are necessary.

3. **Where can I find an accountability partner?**

As cliché as it sounds, my first recommendation is to begin to pray. Keep your eyes open at church. Look for accountability groups online. You can join a Celebrate Recovery in your area. There are many ways to find a partner but the one thing that I recommend is that you do not have a preset notion of what you need in a partner. Because of my brokenness, I would not have picked the people God picked for me. But they were exactly what I needed. God knows what you need. Part of what you need on this journey is accountability, and because you need it, God will provide it. (We will be talking about apps and other resources in the following sections of this chapter.)

4. **What are practical ways I can put accountability in effect?**

One practical way to put accountability into effect is to check in with your partner regarding the habit you desire to change. For example, if you're trying to break a habit, have a predetermined time set aside that you will check in with one another (Number 5 addresses this in more detail). This can be as simple as a thumbs up at the end of the day via text. Also, I recommend being accountable for your behavior and some of the thoughts behind the behavior. For example, I recommend that you have time set aside for someone to ask you questions that the two of you agreed upon, especially at the beginning of accountability. Another practical way to engage in accountability is to have someone ask you questions after you have a slip in your behavior. Also, coming up with an idea concerning what you will do when tempted is helpful, as is being asked why you didn't follow through with those ideas if you engage in the temptation.

5. **How often should I be accountable?**

   That truly is up to you. When deciding this, a couple of things to consider are how often you engage in your unhealthy habit and how much help you feel you need to stop. I have some clients who are accountable every day, some who are accountable several times a week, and some who are accountable once a week. If you're trying to break a habit, I do not recommend being accountable less than once a week. Also, you mustn't be vague but specific regarding your accountability. For example, if you are going to check in with someone once a week, do not just say I will check in with you once a week. Instead, say I will check in with you on Saturdays at 7pm. The same principle applies if you're going to check in every day; let them know you'll be checking in via text in the evening. Let them know what to do if they don't hear from you. If you say you will check in with someone three days a week, let them know the exact days and times. The "perfect" accountability plan, is the one you will stick with.

6. **Should we meet in person or over the phone?**

   I think that either is fine. But, again, it really depends upon you and your schedule. The beautiful thing about the time we live in is that we have many ways to connect. We can connect over zoom, connect over the phone, connect via text, and other ways. So it's more important that we are connecting and that when we do connect, we connect vulnerably and transparently. That being said, I do recognize that there is value in connecting in person. So I do recommend connecting in person, at least on occasion, if possible.

7. **I've already tried it, but it doesn't work. What am I doing wrong?**

   Frequently it's not that accountability doesn't work; it's that we stopped working our accountability. Some become fearful because they had what they perceived to be a bad accountability experience, so they don't want to try again. But what I found most frequently is that when accountability fails, it's not because the other person doesn't want to help. It's actually because accountability wasn't clearly communicated. So, my suggestion is to make sure that everything is clearly communicated, including expectations. Then, take the risk of trying again. The reward of finding the correct person far outweighs the risk.

8. **I'm prone to lying and covering up. How can I make accountability work for me?**

   Of course, it's only up to you whether or not you want to be honest. No one can make you do this. However, something that might help you, and I've seen many people (including myself) utilize, is remembering your tendency when planning your accountability with your partner. You can do this by including questions about your forthrightness: "Are you being honest?" "Are you trying to hide anything?" "Is there anything you ought to be sharing that you are not?"

9. **I find it hard to trust people. What can I do?**

   As was mentioned earlier in this book, it was in relationships you were broken; it is in relationships that you will be healed. I know that it's hard to trust people sometimes. But anything worthwhile takes a challenge. I know it's easier said than done, but take that risk and simply step out and watch what God will do. Start with people you know are very safe, and slowly begin to let others in.

10. Should I keep being accountable if I just keep falling?

Yes. Talk to your accountability partner and see if there's something that you need to change about your accountability. Perhaps stricter consequences for yourself may be beneficial or greater discipline. Don't quit, but perhaps reevaluate.

11. What should I do if my accountability partner doesn't follow through?

Follow through with them and revisit the conversation. Give them permission to back out if they need to and let them know that you understand. If the accountability partner doesn't work, it's time to begin praying and looking for a new one.

12. How long should I be accountable?

I have been accountable to people since I started breaking free from my habits, and I plan on being accountable to people until the day I die. I think we need accountability until we're perfect and we're not going to be perfect in this life.

13. Can I have more than one accountability partner?

Absolutely. It takes stress off of other accountability partners, and it also allows you to not feel pressure when you can't reach someone. But relax, and just start with one.

14. Does my accountability have to always stay the same?

Absolutely not. Your accountability may change as you change and as you grow. So don't get stuck by thinking it has to continue to look the same. Accountability often looks different at each stage of the process.

15. I am really worried that I will bother people, and I hate to be a bother. What should I do?

Dare to believe people when they tell you you're not a bother. If they tell you they want to help you, gird up the loins of your mind and believe that this person is not a liar. Before you even begin the accountability process, ask them if you are being a bother and tell them that they can set any boundaries with you. If they don't let you know anything needs to change, assume that everything is fine. If you suspect that they aren't voicing it or that something is bothering them, simply ask them. It's helpful also to remind yourself that you wouldn't mind helping a friend in need, and they likely are no different.

16. Having accountability seems like a lot of work and is difficult. Why would I want to do this?

It's true. Accountability is not easy. But neither is walking in our addiction or living an incomplete life. We get to choose our difficult. We can choose a difficult that bears good fruit, or we can choose a difficult that leads to destruction. Accountability is a difficulty that bears good fruit.

17. What questions should I ask?

See Chapter Four for sample questions. Truly this is up to what you think and what's going on with you. Remember you are the expert in you. Just because you are broken, like we all are, doesn't mean you don't know what you need. There is no right or wrong concerning the questions. Clear communication is more important than what questions you're going to ask. Also, don't be afraid to tweak your questions as you go along the way.

Software and Apps:

These can serve as a tool for yourself and allow you to share your progress with someone else. These tools should be considered only in addition to accountability with people and not instead of. As always, these are never fail-proof. So, more importantly than having software is having the want to.

These are just a few of the hundreds and perhaps thousands of accountability options available online and/or through Android or iPhones:

Pornography Accountability: Covenant Eyes, Bark, Breathe by Qustodio, Truple, X3Watch, EverAccountable, Accountable2U

Food and Fitness Accountability: 8fit, Body by Blogilates, MyFitnessPal, Streaks Workout, Stacked, Charity Miles, Fooducate

Financial Accountability: YNAB, Mint, Personal Capital, Empower, PocketGuard

General Accountability: StickK, Beeminder, Pact, Goals on Track, HabitShare

Accountability Coach App: Coach.me

Paid Accountability Coach:

This is a great option while you're looking for an accountability partner, or even in addition to one. An accountability coach helps you develop the skills and knowledge that you need to manage your habits and goals to bring positive changes to your activities. A coach can help identify problem areas, create a strategy, define long-term goals and give clarity and direction.

I can provide this type of coaching through my contact page on https://www.divineid.org/contact.html. There are hundreds and hundreds of coaches out there. I am not comfortable recommending any that I do not know personally, but I am happy to provide those I have used.

My business, organizational (and so much more) coach is Rob Stoppard. You can learn more about him at Destinyui.com

My health, weight loss, and fitness coach is Lindsey House. You can learn more about Lindsey at healthaccountabilitycoach.com

> **Questions to ponder:**
>
> Do I see the benefits of practicing some or all of these ways of being accountable? If so, what steps will I take toward making that a reality?

CHAPTER 4

SAMPLE ACCOUNTABILITY QUESTIONS

Please remember these are intended to be only examples. They're not necessarily meant to be followed literally. They're provided to help you get started as you think about what you need for your particular situation. A big part of being accountable is taking the time to recognize patterns that need to be changed. We don't just want to stop the behavior, but we want to recognize what leads or led to that behavior and eliminate that as well.

Some of the things that we utilize accountability for are: stopping a habit, obtaining a goal, starting a habit, and maintaining good habits.

Example of stopping a habit:

(In this case, we will use porn, but of course, you can modify according to whatever habit you're trying to stop)

1. Did you engage in viewing pornography this week? If yes, why didn't you follow the plan you have in place concerning what to do when tempted? What triggered you? What did you learn from your slip? And what will you do differently next time?

2. Did you engage in any borderline behaviors this week? Examples: staying on the internet too long, letting your thoughts take you places they

should not have, going to questionable places (whether in person or online)?

3. Have you been deliberate about connecting with others in healthy intimate ways to combat your need for false intimacy?

4. Have you been intentionally taking relational risks with yourself, God and others?

5. Is there anything you have not shared that I or someone who wants to help you might find concerning?

6. Do you remember why you were doing this?

7. What victories would you like to share?

8. Are you being honest?

9. Is this working? Do we need to change anything?

10. Is there anything else I can do to help?

Obtaining a goal:

(For this example, we will use writing a book)

1. Did you stick with your plan to spend six hours writing this week? If not, why not?

2. Are there any distractions you need to eliminate?

3. Is the weekly goal you have set for yourself realistic?

4. Are there any changes you need to make in adjusting your goal?

5. What barriers have you noticed?

6. Is there anything more I can do to help you obtain this goal?

7. Are there any changes you need to make in your goals or our follow-up?

Starting a new habit:

(We will use being deliberate toward better financial practices.)

1. Have you been keeping up with the budget you planned? If not, why not?

2. Are you being deliberate about placing the designated amount in savings? If not, why not?

3. Have you noticed any patterns in your spending that you'd like to improve?

4. What are your specific goals in this area for the upcoming week?

5. Remind yourself and me why this is important to you?

6. What specific victories have you noticed this week because you're more disciplined in this area?

Maintaining good habits:

(We will use maintaining healthy spiritual habits).

1. Are you being deliberate about connecting with the Lord? If yes, how? If not, what could you do better, and what were your obstacles?

2. Are you watching what you put before your eyes? Please elaborate.

3. In what ways are you being deliberate about serving your spouse and children?

4. Has God been speaking anything to you? And if so, are you being obedient? Are you being deliberate?

5. Are you being deliberate about fighting against legalism in your Christian devotions?

6. Are there any other areas you need to work on?

7. What victories have you experienced in your walk with Christ since we last spoke?

Obviously, this list is not all inconclusive. However, there are countless ways that accountability can be utilized.

Remember, it's not about doing it perfectly. It really is about just taking steps to do it and then committing to it. So, I hope that with this chapter and the previous, you will have a good starting point for your accountability journey.

> **Questions to ponder:**
>
> What type of accountability do I specifically need, and what specific questions would benefit me? When will I schedule a time to complete this important task?

CHAPTER 5

A CALL TO ACTION

Congratulations, you've made it this far and worked your way through the meat of the book. By now, my guess is that you can see the benefits of accountability. But, if you're still not convinced or perhaps just in need of some additional motivation, feel free to go back and review some of the testimonies in Chapter One.

Let's revisit our questions to ponder from the previous chapters, along with some encouragement if you still need to take these steps.

Chapter One:
What goals could be achieved a year from now if I implemented this type of accountability today?

The possibilities for an improved life are endless. Weight loss, financial gain, ending of a poor habit, beginning good habits, etc.

Chapter Two:
While keeping James 5:16 in mind, "Confess your faults one to another and pray for one another, that you may be healed." Ask yourself: What may still need healing in my life because I haven't involved others in my journey?

Take the time to ask God what He wants to heal and who He wants to bring in your life for an accountability partner. A life of wholeness and healing awaits you.

Chapter Three:
Do I see the benefits of practicing some or all of these ways of being accountable? If so, what steps will I take toward making that a reality?

Take whatever practical steps you still need to make this a reality. For help remembering some of the how-tos, see chapters two and three.

Chapter Four:
What type of accountability do I specifically need, and what specific questions would benefit me?
When will I schedule the time to complete this important task?

If you haven't done so, take the time to write out some questions. If you can't do it now, then set a time in your calendar to do this.

My desire for you is to find freedom in every area of your life. From my own experience and the experiences of hundreds I have counseled, I know that accountability is key in making changes happen. I desire for you the courage to implement the things discussed in this book. As good as the idea of accountability is, it can't work if it isn't implemented. So, go for it.

I wish to leave you with this prayer:

Lord Jesus,

Thank You for the person that is reading this right now. I agree with Your Word, which states that it is for freedom that You have set them free. I pray that You give them a hunger to walk in that freedom. I ask that You give them the strength to do their part while having faith that You have already done Your part when You died for them on Calvary. They already have all they need to live out the freedom You purchased. Lead them and guide them to wise and patient accountability partners. Give them the courage to be honest with themselves and others as they partner with You on this journey. Amaze them at what You can do. I bless them and leave them in Your very loving hands.

Amen.

EPILOGUE

ACCOUNTABILITY QUOTES

1. Accountability breeds response-ability.

   - Stephen R. Covey

2. A body of men holding themselves accountable to nobody ought not to be trusted by anybody.

   - Thomas Paine

3. Accountability separates the wishes in life from the action takers that care enough about their future to account for their daily actions.

   - John Di Lemme

4. Accountability is the measure of a leader's height.

   - Jeffrey Benjamin

5. Good men are bound by conscious and liberated by accountability.

   - Wes Fessler

6. Anyone can possess, anyone can profess, but it is an altogether different thing to confess.

   - Shannon L Alder

7. You steadily grow into becoming your best as you choose to be accountable and accept responsibility for improvement.

   - Steve Shallenberger

8. For most people blaming others is a subconscious mechanism for avoiding accountability. In reality, the only thing in your way is you.

   - Steve Maraboli

9. On one side of accountability is courage, on the other side is freedom.

   - Jean Hamilton Ford

10. To be accountable means that we are willing to be responsible to another person for our behavior and it implies a level of submission to another person's opinions and viewpoints.

    - Wayne Goodall

11. Accountability is a statement of personal promise, both to yourself and the people around you to deliver specific, defined results.

    - Brian Dive

12. The time has come to carry accountability forward, to make it offline and into the real world. To share our lives with just a few people we really truly honestly trust.

    - Craig gross

13. The benefits and possibilities that are created by being personally accountable are countless.

- Jay Fiset

14. If you try to take on changes on your own, it is easy not to keep yourself accountable. Try telling a close friend or family member what you're doing and have them check in on you periodically.

- Kathy Stanton

15. Jesus understood the value of relationships, teamwork and accountability. Effective ministry often erupts from small teams.

- Beth Beutler

16. It means a lot. It means I'm accountable.

- Champ Bailey

17. I believe that accountability is the basis of all meaningful human achievement.

- Sam Silverstein.

18. To be accountable or to be a victim is one of those elemental decisions that everyone needs to make. Simply the former leads you to a happier and more rewarding life.

- Rob Pitfield

19. Accountability to others and for what you do begins with respect for who you are and your behavior.

- Byron Pulsifer

20. One of the biggest lessons I've learned about habit development is that you need accountability to stick to a major goal. It's not enough to make a personal commitment.

- S. J. Scott

21. Good Men prefer to be accountable.

- Michael Edwardes

22. Where there is no accountability there will also be no responsibility.

- Sunday Angela

23. When accountability is present, people keep their eyes on a very clear prize. They know what they're working toward and how they're going to get there.

- Henry J. Evans

24. True Love does not only encompass the things that make you feel good, it also holds you to a standard of accountability.

- Monica Johnson

25. Accountability is the glue that ties the commitment to the result.

- Bob Proctor

Made in the USA
Columbia, SC
21 September 2024